NATURAL HAIR AND SKINCARE REMEDIES
(VOLUME II: SKIN REMEDIES)

By
Brittany M Robinson

Natural Hair And Skin Care Remedies

(Volume II: Skin Remedies)

Copyright © 2022 by Brittany M Robinson

Published By: Brittany M Robinson

Printed in the United States of America

ISBN: 979-8-9862607-2-3 (Hardcover)
979-8-9862607-5-4 (Paperback)

For information Contact:

Mrs. Robinson Natural Solutions at Https://

mrsrobinsonnaturalsolutions.com

All natural products to make your hair healthier and grow faster. Keep your hair healthy by using natural products. Butter and oil are healthy for your hair and body.

A little about me— I'm a happily married Mother of 4. I got the inspiration for my book from my children.

Skin and body rash is sometime an inflammation of the skin. You might see a change in the color of the skin or texture. Rashes could irritate the skin or cause an allergic reaction. Allergies could be due to food, plants, chemicals, animals, insects, and the environmental. Skin rash could affect the entire body or area of the body. Eruptions on the skin of the back are called Back Rash. Even though All rashes are not contagious, some could be.

One day, I noticed my son, JerMichael, had got some rashes; I used different types of products for a few months, but it didn't help. The rashes on his body were very serious, and the doctor said that we should not apply any products without knowing what is in the products. It can put your children in great danger of skin-related issues. After that, I studied it, and I believe there are many people out there who are facing the same issue.

After spending thousands of dollars on different products, this book includes all the tips and steps I tried in getting rid of my son's rashes. If you purchase this book, you can save thousands of dollars or hundreds of hours, as I've wasted mine to help you. I started making my natural body wash, oils, butter, and body pain oils. The rash you are experiencing may have a different root than my son's. However, I believe this book can help you.

Note:

If you on any medication or pregnant consult with your doctor.

Table of Contents

Mango Butter Cream

Ingredients:

- 2 Tbs. Beeswax
- 2 Tbs. Mango butter
- 8 Tbs. Coconut oil
  10 drops carrot seed essential oil

Directions:

1. Melt wax and butter in a double boiler.
2. Add oil, keep stirring it, allow it to cool, let it harden, and blend it.
3. Add essential oils and keep mixing them until the mixture is completely smooth.
4. Pour into a jar and let it harden. (Mango butter also reduces degeneration of skin cells and restores elasticity).

Kokum & Tucuma Chocolate Butter

Ingredients:

- 3 oz Kokum Butter
- 2 oz Tucuma Butter
- 3 oz Jojoba oil
- 3 tsp argan oil
- 1tsp cocoa powder
- 10 -20 drops vanilla essential oil

Directions:

1. Melt butter in a double boil.
2. Put it in the refrigerator until it's solid.
3. Add oils and cocoa powder. Use a hand mixer until it becomes creamy.
4. Add essential oils and mix it until smooth.
5. Pour it into a jar.

Shea Butter Cream

Ingredients:

- 2 Tbs. Beeswax
- 2 Tbs. Shea butter
- 8 Tbs. sunflower oil
- 1tsp Vitamins E

Directions:

1. Melt wax and butter in a double boiler.
2. Add oil, and keep stirring it.
3. Allow it to cool, let it harden, and then blend it.
4. Add essential oils and keep mixing them until the mixture is completely smooth.
5. Pour it into a jar and let it harden.

Cocoa Butter and vanilla Cream

Ingredients:

- 2 Tbs. Beeswax
- 2 Tbs. cocoa butter butter
- 4 Tbs. sunflower oil
- 4 Tbs. Borage oil
- 1tsp Vitamins E

Directions:

1. Melt wax and butter in a double boiler.
2. Add oil, and keep stirring it.
3. Allow it to cool, let it harden, and then blend it.
4. Add essential oils and keep mixing them until the mixture is completely smooth.
5. Pour it into a jar and let it harden.

Shea Butter and Aloe vera Cream

Ingredients:

- 2 Tbs. carnauba wax
- 2 Tbs. Shea butter
- 8 Tbs. argan oil
- 2 Tbs. Aloe vera
- 1tsp Vitamins E

Directions:

1. Melt wax and butter in a double boiler.
2. Add oil and aloe vera; keep stirring it, allow it to cool, let it harden, and blend it.
3. Add essential oils and keep mixing them until the mixture is completely smooth.
4. Pour it into a jar and let it harden.

Ayurvedic butter

Ingredients:

- 2 Tbs. Ayurvedic butter
- 8 Tbs. argan oil
- 2 Tbs. Mango butter
- 1tsp Vitamins E
- 10 drops lemongrass essential oil
- 10 drops cedarwood essential oil

Directions:

1. Melt butter in a double boiler.
2. Add oil, keep stirring it, allow it to cool, let it harden, and blend it.
3. Add essential oils and keep mixing them until the mixture is completely smooth.
4. Pour it into a jar and let it harden.

Blueberry & vanilla Face mist

Ingredients:

- 2 ½ cup Distilled water
- 7 drop vanilla
- 7 drop blueberry

Directions:

1. Put your blueberries and water in the pot, then put the steamer basket inside your pot on top of your blueberries.
2. Now put the heatproof bowl inside and put your lid upside down, so you can collect the water. Keep it for 1 hour (you are making Hydrosol).
3. Put a lot of ice in a bag on top of your lid.
4. Then pour the water into the jar and add 7 drops vanilla.

Chamomile Mist for skin

Ingredients:

- 2 1/2 cup Distill Water
- 2tsp Chamomile

Directions:

1. Put your flowers and water in the pot, then put the steamer basket inside your pot on top of your flowers and water, then place a heat-proof bowl inside and place the lid upside down for 1 hour (you are making Hydrosol).
2. Put a lot of ice in a bag on top of your lid.
3. Put it in a container.

Hibiscus Flowers Mist for skin

Ingredients:

- 2 ½ cup Distilled water
- 2tsp Hibiscus flowers (dried)
- 2tsp rose petals

Direction:

1. Put your flowers and water in the pot, put the steamer basket inside your pot on top of your flowers and water, then place a heatproof bowl inside, and place the lid upside down for 1 hour (you are making Hydrosol).
2. Put a lot of ice in a bag on top of your lid.
3. Put it into a container.

Blueberry & Apple Mist for skin

Ingredients:

- 3 ½ cups distilled Water
- 5 apples
- 1 cup berries

Directions:

1. Put your blueberries, apples, and water in the pot, then put the steamer basket inside your pot on top of your blueberries and apples.
2. Now put the heatproof bowl inside and put your lid upside down so you can collect the water for 1 hour (you are making Hydrosol).
3. Put a lot of ice in a bag on top of your lid.
4. Then pour the water into the jar.

Apples and orange Mist for skin

Ingredients:

- 3 ½ cups distilled Water
- 4 apples cut up
- 4 oranges cut up

Directions:

1. Put your (cut up) oranges and apples and water in the pot, then put the steamer basket inside your pot on top of your oranges and apples.
2. Now put the heatproof bowl inside and put your lid upside down so you can collect the water for 1 hour (you are making Hydrosol).
3. Put a lot of ice in a bag on top of your lid.
4. Then pour the water into the jar

Basil Mist for skin

Ingredients:

- 3 ½ cups distilled Water
- 20 Basil

Directions:

1. Put your basil and water in the pot, then put the steamer basket inside your pot on top of your basil.
2. Now put the heatproof bowl inside, and put your lid upside down so you can collect the water. Low heat for 1 hour (you are making Hydrosol).
3. Put a lot of ice in a bag on top of your lid.
4. Then pour the water into the spray bottle and add 7 drops Geranium.

Green tea & cucumber for skin Mist

Ingredients:

- 3 ½ cups distilled Water
- 4 cucumber
- 2 bags of green tea

Directions:

1. Put your cucumber, green tea, and water in the pot, then put the steamer basket inside your pot on top of your cucumber and green tea.
2. Now put the heatproof bowl inside and put your lid upside down so you can collect the water. Low eat for 1 hour (you are making Hydrosol).
3. Put a lot of ice in a bag on top of your lid.
4. Then pour the water into the spray bottle.

Lavender & Sage for skin Mist

Ingredients:

- 3 ½ cups distilled Water
- 2tsp lavender leaves
- 2tsp sage

Directions:

1. Put your sage, lavender, and water in the pot, then put the steamer basket inside your pot on top of your sage and lavender.
2. Now put the heatproof bowl inside and put your lid upside down so you can collect the water. Low eat for 1 hour (you are making Hydrosol).
3. Put a lot of ice in a bag on top of your lid.
4. Then pour the water into the spray bottle.

Bergamot Mist for skin

Ingredients:

- 2 1/2 cup Distill Water
- 1 tsp bergamot
- 1 tsp vanilla

Direction:

1. Put your bergamot, vanilla, and water in the pot, then put the steamer basket inside your pot on top of your beragmot, vanilla, and water.
2. Then place a heatproof bowl inside and place the lid upside down for 1 hour (you are making Hydrosol).
3. Put a lot of ice in a bag on top of your lid.
4. Put it in a container.

Lime and Lemon Mist for skin

Ingredients:

- 3 ½ cups distilled Water
- 4 lemons
- 4 limes
- 2 tsp honey

Directions:

1. Put your lemons, lime, honey, and water in the pot, then put the steamer basket inside your pot on top of your lemons, lime, and honey
2. Put the heatproof bowl inside and put your lid upside down so you can collect the water. Low eat for 1 hour (you are making Hydrosol).
3. Put a lot of ice in a bag on top of your lid.
4. Then pour the water into the spray bottle.

Orange and lavender Body Spray

Ingredients:

- 8oz cups distilled Water
- 2oz Perfumery Alcohol
- 2oz witch hazel
- 1 tsp glycerin
- 7 drops lavender

Directions:

1. Stir it until well-combined.
2. Pour it into a bottle.
3. Add fragrance of sweet orange and lavender.
4. You can add orange peels (make sure the peels dry).

Pink strawberry Body Spray

Ingredients:

- 8oz cups distilled Water
- 2oz Perfumery Alcohol
- 2oz witch hazel
- 1 tsp glycerin
- 0.15oz strawberry fragrance
- 0.15oz Pink sugar fragrance

Directions:

1. Stir ingredients until mixed.
2. Pour it into a bottle.
3. Add fragrance.

Star Jasmine and sweet Spray perfume

Ingredients:

- 18 ml Distilled Water
- 4 ml Polysorbate 80
- 16 ml organic Alcohol or 96% alcohol
- 1 oz Fragrance Oil Blend (Star Jasmine, sweet orange)
- 0.5 ml Optiphen

Directions:

- Keep stirring it until mixed well.
- Put it into a spray bottle.

Natural Perfume Oil

Ingredients:

- 16g Borage oil
- 4g essential oi fragrance blend
- 1g Vitamin E oil
- 30 drops vanilla essential oil
- 15 drops rosemary essential oil
- 4 drops sweet orange essential oil
- 6 drops bergamot

Directions:

1. Put all ingredients in a pot, and mix them.
2. Pour it into a spray container.

Spray perfume

Ingredients:

- 18 ml Distilled Water
- 4 ml Polysorbate 80
- 16 ml organic Alcohol or 96% alcohol
- 1 oz Fragrance Oil Blend (Star Jasmine, sweet orange)
- 0.5 ml Optiphen

Directions:

1. Keep stirring it until it turns clear.

3. Put it in a spray bottle.

Natural Perfume Oil

Ingredients:

- 16g Borage oil
- 4g essential oi fragrance blend
- 1g Vitamin E oil
- 15 drops vanilla essential oil
- 15 drops rose essential oil
- 12 drops cinnamon essential
- 7 drops lemon essential oil
- 4 drops bergamot

Directions:

1. Put all ingredients in the measured and mix, then pour it into a container.

Solid Perfume

Ingredients:

- 1.6 oz Sunflower
- 1.2 oz White Beeswax
- 0.5 oz jojoba
- 0.7 oz Meadowfoam oil
- 1 oz Essential oil (Rose quartz fragrance)

Directions:

1. Get a glass heat bowl; you can put it in the microwave until it melts.
2. Stir it, then put it in the lip-balm container.

Sunflower Skin cream

Ingredients:

- 80g Distilled water
- 1g colloidal oatmeal
- 2g honey
- 2g Shea Butter
- 5g Emulsifying wax
- 1g sunflower

Directions:

1. Water Distilled, then add honey and colloidal oatmeal.
2. Use a hand blender until it mixes together.
3. Put the Shea butter, emulsify wax, and sunflower in a separate container.
4. Put water in a pot with a glass container. Keep stirring butter until it melts, then add distilled water ingredients until it mixes.
5. Then take it out of the heat.
6. Use a hand mixer until thick.
7. Add 1g vitamin E oil.
8. Add 7 drop vanilla oil.
9. 2% add natural Preservative (10 drops grapefruit oil).

10. Put it in a container.

Skin cream

Ingredients:

- 1 cups rose hip oil
- 1 cup of aloe vera juice
- 1/3 cup Emulsifying wax
- 3tbs of cocoa butter
- 6 tsp of honey or vegetable glycerin
- 7 drop rosemary oil
- 7 drop vanilla oil
- 2% Leucidal liquid SF

Directions:

1. Put the oils and waxes in a pot on low heat until they melt.
2. Then remove it from the heat.
3. Use your hand mixer, start mixing it, then add the Aloe vera juice and vegetable glycerin slowly.
4. Add 7 drops vanilla, rosemary oil, and add Leucidal liquid SF.

Carrot and cranberry cream for glowing skin

Ingredients:

- 2 carrots
- ½ cup Aloe vera
- ½ cup borage oil
- 2% Leucidal liquid SF
- 10 drops cranberry seed oil

Directions:

1. Grate the carrots dry and put them in the microwave for 2 min.
2. Put a pot of water on the stove (heat low).
3. Put the carrots and oil in a glass container, then put the glass in the water until the oil changes color.
4. Then remove it from the heat (let it cool).
5. Add aloe vera.
6. Use your hand mixer until it becomes smooth.
7. Put it in a container.
8. Add 10 drops cranberry seed oil and Leucidal liquid SF.

Rosewater moisturizer

Ingredients:

- 6.4 oz Rosewater
- 0.4 oz Glycerin Colloidal Oatmeal
- 0.07 oz Avocado Butter
- 0.17 oz pomegranate oil
- o.17 oz avocado oil
- 0.17 oz jojoba oil
- 0.5oz Emulsifying Wax
- 0.4 oz Leucidal Liquid SF (natural Preservative)
- 0.07 oz Honey
- 0.07 oz Vitamin E oil (Antioxidant)
- 10 drops rosemary essential oils

Directions:

1. Use a double boiler on low heat, then add avocado butter and let it melt, and add water and olive oil.
2. Add oils and emulsifying wax and keep stirring it, then add glycerin & colloidal oatmeal. Let it sit and cool down. Whip the mixture up with a hand mixer.
3. It will look creamy, then add your natural Leucidal, honey, Vitamins E, and Essential oils.
4. It is ready to store in a container or pump bottle.

Shea Butter moisturizer

Ingredients:

- 8 oz raw, unrefined Shea Butter
- 1 tsp Jojoba Oil
- 1tsp honey
- 5 drops spearmint Essential oil
- 5 drops lemongrass essential oil
- 5 drops rosemary essential oil

Directions:

1. Use a double boiler and add Shea butter and jojoba oil to a bowl.
2. Add 5 drops spearmint and lemongrass essential oil.
3. Then get it off the double boiler, let it cool, then whip the mixture up with a hand mixer.
4. Pour it into a container.

Rosewater Body Wash

Ingredients:

- 1 cup liquid Castile soap
- 2tsp vegetable glycerin
- 1/2 cup rosewater
- 1tsp jojoba oil
- 1tsp baking soda
- ¼ cup raw honey
- 15 rosemary essential oil or (lemongrass)
- 5 drops Bulgarian rose essential oil
- 1tsp vitamin E
- 1tsp tea tree

Directions:

1. Put all the ingredients in the pump bottle.
2. Shake the ingredients in the bottle to combine them.
3. Add Essential oil (option).
4. Ready to use.

Body wash

Ingredients:

- 1/2 cup Hibiscus or cucumber water
- ½ cup honey
- 2 tsp castor oil
- 2tsp jojoba oil
- 2tsp castile soap
- 1tsp neem oil
- 1/3 cup alcohol-free witch hazel
- 10drops vanilla essential oil
- 5 drops orange essential oil
- 5 drops thyme essential oil
- 5 drops Mandarin essential oil or Juniper berry oil

Directions:

1. Put all the ingredients in the pump bottle.
2. Shake the ingredients in the bottle to combine them.
3. Add Essential oil (option).
4. Ready to use.

Rose and Lemon body wash

Ingredients:

- ½ cup rose water
- ½ cup witch hazel (alcohol-free)
- 2tsp jojoba oil
- 1tsp honey
- 1tsp Castile soap
- 10 lemon drops essential oil

Directions:

1. Put all the ingredients in the pump bottle.
2. Shake the ingredients in the bottle to combine them.
3. Add Essential oil (optional).
4. Ready to use.

Rose Petal Sugar scrub

Ingredients:

- 44g Cocoa Butter
- 14g Almond oil or Argan oil
- ½ g Vitamin E oil
- 6g Candelilla wax
- essential vanilla & lavender
- 6g oats
- 6g Sugar or brown sugar
- ½ g Arrowroot powder
- 1g rose petals
- 10 drops palmarosa oil
- ½ honey

Directions:

1. Melt butter and oil, then put wax in a double boiler. When mixed together, it will get smooth, then put it in the refrigerator to thicken for 30 minutes.
2. When the mixture cools down, add the Vitamin E. Now add the rose petal and sugar. Keep mixing it, then put it in the soap molds and leave to refrigerate overnight.

Brown Sugar Body Scrub

Ingredients:

- 1 cup olive oil
- 1cup brown sugar
- 1tsp honey
- essential chamomile

Directions:

1. Combine oil and sugar, then add essential oil and mix it.
2. Store it in the container.

Sea moss for face cream

Directions:

1. Put sea moss into a bowl, then fill it up with spring water and let it sit for 12 hours. You can add lemon or lime as it gives it a natural flavor.
2. Now take it out of the water to blend it up, put your sea moss in the blender, then fill the spring water to the same amount of sea moss you have, or you can add more water if needed. You will see the sea moss jump when blending. Once you are done, it will be smooth.
3. Then put it in the jar.
4. You can apply it to your face daily.
5. Keep it in the refrigerator for two months.

Skin toner cream

Ingredients:

- 1/2cup okra gel
- 2 tsp Beeswax
- ¼ cup Argan oil
- 7 drop lemongrass essential oil

Directions:

1. Melt the Beeswax and oil in a double boiler. Add okra gel and mix with your hand blender.
2. Add essential oil.
3. Put it into a glass container.

Coconut Butter Body Lotion

Ingredients:

- 2 tablespoons Gelatin
- 4 oz. cocoa butter
- 4 tablespoons sweet almond oil or grapeseed oil
- 2 tablespoons argan oil

Directions:

1. Melt the cocoa butter in a double boiler. Add gelatin and oils, stir it or blend it until mixed. Then let it cool down.
2. Pour it into a glass jar.
3. You can add 5 to 10 drops essential oil.
4. The lotion will thicken as it cools.

Eczema Cream Lotion

Ingredients:

- 1 tablespoons beeswax
- 2 oz Cupuacu butter or Shea butter
- 2 tablespoons hemp oil
- 1tsp nutmeg powder
- 10 drops German Chamomile
- 10 drops Lavender
- 10 drops vitamin E oil

Directions:

1. Use a double boiler to melt wax and butter.
2. Add oils and nutmeg powder, and let it cool down.
3. Then use the hand blender to smooth the mixture, and then add essential oil.
4. Put it in a container.

Coconut Lotion

Ingredients:

- 1 cup Coconut oil
- 2tsp Aloe Vera gel
- 1tsp honey
- 5 drops orange essential oil
- 5 drops lavender essential oil

Directions:

1. Use a double boiler for coconut to melt it.
2. Let it cool down.
3. Then use the hand blender to smooth the mixture.
4. Add aloe vera gel, honey, and essential oil, then blend it well.
5. Put it in a container.

Chamomile Body lotion

Ingredients:

- 1/8 tsp baking soda
- ¼ cup chamomile tea
- ½ cup canola or olive oil or sunflower
- 1 tsp grated beeswax
- 1 tsp cocoa butter (dry skin)

Directions:

1. In a saucepan, put chamomile tea and pour the baking soda until dissolved.
2. Use a double boiler (on low flame) to melt wax and butter. Keep stirring it until its completely melt. (It's best to have 2 saucepans).
3. Slowly add baking soda to the mixture while stirring it.
4. Let the lotion cool down. Keep stirring it so the water and oil don't separate.
5. Pour it into a container.

Body lotion sensitive skin

Ingredients:

- ½ tbsp raw honey
- ½ tbsp aloe Vera gel or aloe ferox
- ½ tbsp Cucumber gel
- 3 tbsp Calendula oil
- 10 drops Lavender or chamomile oil
- ½ vitamin E (option)

Directions:

1. Put all your ingredients into a bottle or container, then shake it to combine.
2. Store it in the fridge.

Chocolate &vanilla Lotion Bar recipe

Ingredients:

- 4.5 oz White beeswax
- 3 oz Olive oil or Sweet almond oil
- 3 oz Cocoa butter Wafers
- 1tsp Vanilla fragrance oil(option)
- 1tsp cocoa powder (optional)

Directions:

1. Put the crockpot, and add white beeswax and oil. Stir it until its melted.
2. Add cocoa butter wafers to hot wax and mix it with oil. Keep stirring it until the butter melts.
3. Add Vanilla oil and cocoa powder; keep stirring it.
4. Pour it into the mold and let it harden, and pop them out.

Lavender lotion bar

Ingredients:

- 3 oz Cocoa Butter
- 3 oz jojoba oil
- 4.5 White Beeswax
- ½ tsp Arrowroot powder
- ½ tsp Vitamin E
- 5 drops lavender essential oil or fragrance (optional)

Directions:

1. Put the crockpot, and add white beeswax and oil. Keep stirring it until it's melted. (Optional You can melt it in the microwave for 60 seconds using a suitable container).
2. Add cocoa butter wafers to hot wax and mix it with oil. Keep stirring it until the jojoba oil melts. Add the Vitamin E and Arrowroot powder.
3. Add Lavender essential oil and keep stirring it.
4. Pour it into the mold and allow it to harden, then pop them out.

Rosewater lotion bar

Ingredients:

- 3.6 oz cup cocoa butter
- 1 tsp rosewater
- 3.6 oz White Beeswax
- 2.4 oz Jojoba oil
- Fragrance oil or essential (optional)

Directions:

1. Put the crockpot, add white beeswax and oil; stir it until it melts. (Optional you can melt it in the microwave for 60 seconds. Make sure you have a suitable container).
2. Add cocoa butter wafers to hot wax and mix it with oil. Keep stirring it until the butter melts.
3. Add rosewater and keep stirring it.
4. Pour it into the mold. You can put rose petals in it, allow it to harden, then pop them out.

Rose Geranium Body Oil Recipe

Ingredients:

- 4 oz Apricot Kernel Oil
- 10 drops geranium Essential Oil
- 10 drops Rose Essential Oil
- 10 drops bergamot Essential Oil

Directions:

1. Get a glass (dark), add the oils and shake it up.

Grape-seed Body Oil skin

Ingredients:

- 4 teaspoons Cranberry Oil
- 4 teaspoons Pomegranate Oil
- 4 tablespoon Grape-seed Oil
- 15 drops Carrot Essential oil
- 10 drops Myrrh Essential oil
- 10 drops Neroli Essential oil

Directions:

1. Get a glass bottle (dark) and add the oils, then shake it up.

Lavender Body Oil Recipe

Ingredients:

- 4 oz olive oil
- 10 drops chamomile roman essential oil
- 10 drops lavender essential oil
- 10 drops bergamot essential oil

Directions:

1. Get a glass bottle (dark), add the oils, and shake it up.

Sandalwood Body Oil Recipe

Ingredients:

- 3 oz Jojoba Oil
- 5 drops ylang-ylang essential oils
- 5 drops sandalwood essential oils
- 5 drops patchouli essential oils

Directions:

1. Get a glass bottle (dark), add the oils, and then shake it up.

Mint Vanilla Grape-seed body oil Recipe

Ingredients:

- 4 oz Grape-seed Oil
- 10 drops Essential Oil
- 10 drops Eucalyptus Essential Oil
- 10 drops Peppermint Essential Oil
- 5 drops vanilla oil

Directions:

1. Get a glass bottle (dark), add the oils, and then shake it up.

Basil oil for skin

Ingredients:

- Avocado oil
- Fresh chop basil, 10 small pieces

Directions:

1. Put the pot of water on the stove.
2. Get a small pot so you can put it inside another pot.
3. Put the oil and basil leaves in the small pot.
4. Put the heat on low.
5. Get a spoon, mix it at a boil for 20 minutes.
6. Cover it for the heat, allow it to cool for 4 hours.
7. Then strain out the basil.
8. Pour it into a glass bottle.
9. Apply to your skin.

16 Extra Remedies For free

Toothache oil

Clove essential oil treats toothache oil. A few drops of clove oil can be mixed with warm water, then you can gargle to relieve your throat pain. (Jojoba oil or olive oil) Peppermint, Lavender, cinnamon toothache oil. Put the oils on the areas that are hurt.

Mix with clove oil, massage on the affected area. You will get some relief from muscle, joint pain, and soreness.

Back Pain oil

Ingredients:

- 8 drops rosemary oil
- 9 drops peppermint oil
- 10 lavender oil
- 6 marjoram oil
- 2tsp jojoba oil

Directions:

1. Get a glass container, then shake it all together. Ready to use.
2. Massage your body two times a day.

Bone pain oil

Ingredients:

- 10 myrrh oil
- 6 ginger oil
- 7 orange oil
- 2 tsp jojoba oil

Directions:

1. Get a glass container, then shake it all together. Ready to use.
2. Massage your body 2 times a day.

Sinus pain oil

Ingredients:

- 3 drops rosemary oil
- 3 drops peppermint oil

Directions:

1. Boil water, pour it into a large bowl, and add oil.
2. Inhale the mixture for 10 minutes.

Swelling reduce oil

Ingredients:

- 5 drops Lemongrass oil
- 5 drops ginger oil
- 5 drops lavender oil
- 5 drops Helichrysum oil
- 2 drops Eucalyptus oil
- 2 drops Lavender oil
- 2tsp olive oil

Directions:

1. Get a glass container, then shake it all together. Ready to use.
2. Massage your body 2 times a day.

Cancer treatment pain oil

Ingredients:

- 6 drops Lemongrass oil
- 5 drops Myrrh oil
- 5 drops Peppermint oil
- 3 drops Spearmint oil
- 2 drops Frankincense oil
- 2tsp olive oil

Directions:

1. Get a glass container, then shake it all together. Ready to use.
2. Massage your body 2 times a day.

Leg restless oil

Ingredients:

- 4 drops Marjoram oil
- 4 drops Lemongrass oil
- 4 drops peppermint oil
- 2tsp olive oil

Directions:

1. Put it in a container, then shake it all together. It is time to use it.
2. Massage your body or put it in a warm bath 2 times a day.

Fever oil

1. Rosemary oil is effective as it is anti-inflammatory, inhale the vapors so you can relieve your headache.
2. Peppermint is also great and can help relieve headaches and sinus congestion.
3. You can apply it on your forehead or back of your neck a few times a day.

Muscle Relaxation oil

Ingredients:

- 3 lavender oil
- 3 Chamomile oil
- 3 peppermint oil
- 3 Thyme oil
- Olive oil or grade seed oil

Directions:

1. Get a glass container, then shake it all together. Ready to use.
2. Massage your body 2 times a day.

Pain oil

Ingredients:

- 7 drops Peppermint oil
- 7 drops geranium oil
- 7 drops ginger oil
- 7 drops lavenders oil
- 7 drops eucalyptus oil
- 5 drops Juniper
- 2tsp castor oil

Directions:

1. Get a glass container, then shake it all together.
2. Ready to use. Massage your body 2 times a day.

Menstruation & cramps pain reliever oil

Ingredients:

- 2tsp coconut oil or Olive oil
- 5drops neem oil
- 5drops peppermint oil
- 5 drops eucalyptus oil
- 5 drops lavender oil
- 5 drops clary sage oil
- 5drops Ylang-Ylang oil or clove oil

Directions:

1. Put all these oils in a bottle, then shake it up.
2. Apply it to the pain area.

Menstruation pain reliever oil

Ingredients:

- 2 tsp ginger oil
- 5 drops frankincense oil
- 5 drops mustard oil
- 5 Chamomile oil
- 5drops cinnamon oil
- 5 drops lemon oil

Directions:

1. Put all these oils in a bottle, then shake.
2. Apply it to the pain area.

Spider Vein pain oil

Ingredients:

- 10 drops Geranium oil
- 10 drops cypress oil
- 5 drops peppermint oil
- 5 drops lemon oil
- 5 drops lavender oil
- 2 tsp olive oil or castor oil
- 5 drops Clary Sage If you have swelling it will reduce with this oil (option)

Directions:

1. Get a glass container, then shake it all together. Ready to use.
2. Massage your body 2 times a day.

Lose weight oil

Ingredients:

- 10 Peppermint oil
- 10 grapefruit oil
- 10 Ginger oil
- 5 Cinnamon oil
- 2tsp castor oil or olive oil

Directions:

1. Put it in a container, then shake it all together. It is time to use it.
2. Massage your body 2 times a day. It will boost up your metabolism and you will lose weight. Exercise will also be helpful.

Stress oil

Ingredients:

- 4 drops lavender oil
- 4 drops lime oil
- 2 drops spearmint oil
- 1 tsp castor oil

Directions:

1. Get a glass container, then shake it all together. Ready to use.
2. Massage your body 2 times a day.

Vaginal Hygiene

1. Have a healthy diet - put in pears, pineapples, melons, dates, bananas, coconut, or green coconut water. (It will help with Heavy Menstruation).

2. When on your menstruation, you should eat more calcium and iron-rich foods because you lose a lot of blood during your menstruation. It will light up your menstruation and give you a better smell down there.

3. Eating wheat germ oil, sunflower, and pumpkin seed will help with ovulation.

4. Eating yogurt and drinking buttermilk ½ cup every morning and night will help decrease yeast.

5. Drink ginger and green tea while adding honey, cinnamon, turmeric, and little cloves to it.

6. You can soak Coriander seeds with water overnight, then strain in the morning and drink it. It removes all toxins from the body.

7. Mix coconut oil and a few drops of neem oil, and apply to the vagina area to relieve pain (itching or burning).

These are natural preservatives - rosemary, jojoba, grapefruit seed oil, rosemary extract, citric acid, lemon juice, Leucidal liquid SF and sugar. Add in your product to make them last longer.

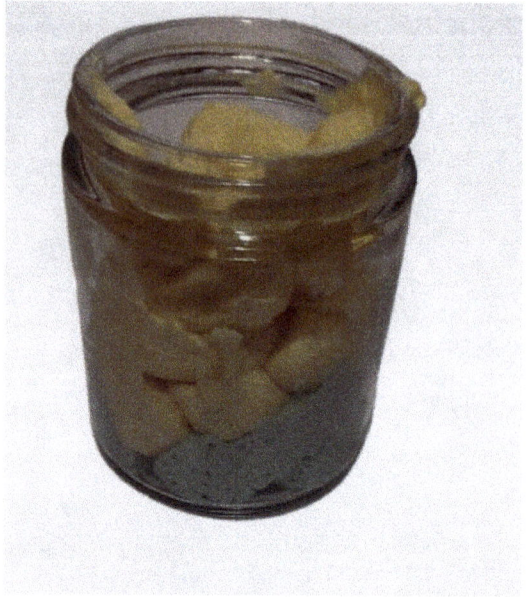

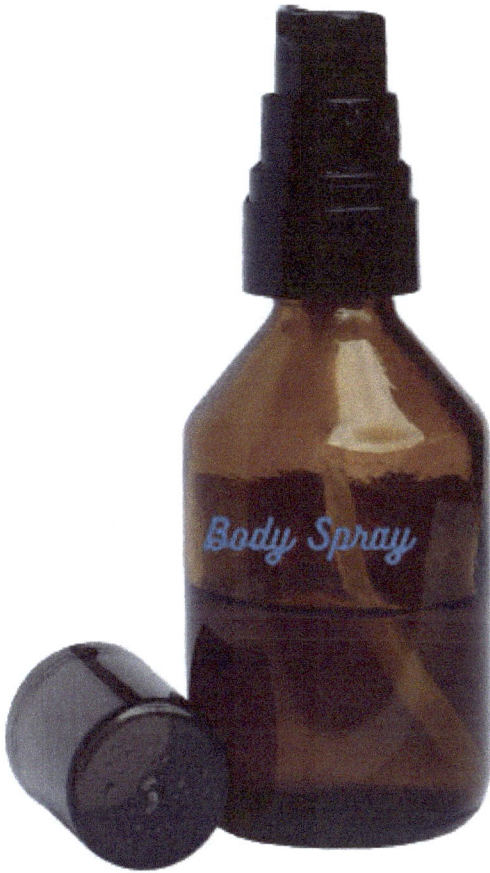

www.ingramcontent.com/pod-product-compliance
Lightning Source LLC
Chambersburg PA
CBHW050217270326
41914CB00003BA/447